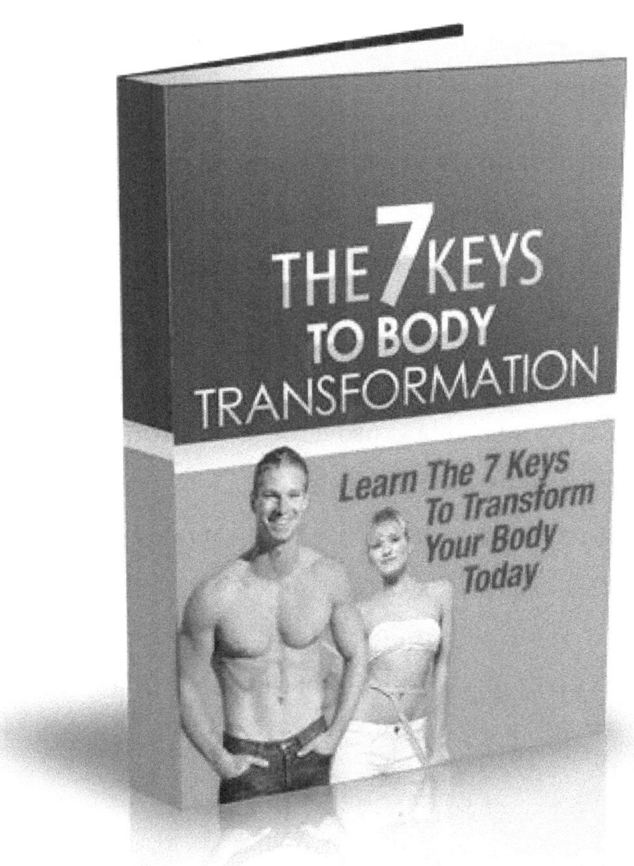
THE 7 KEYS
TO BODY
TRANSFORMATION
Learn The 7 Keys
To Transform
Your Body
Today

Copyright © 2013

Disclaimer

All the material contained in this book is provided for educational and informational purposes only. No responsibility can be taken for any results or outcomes resulting from the use of this material. While every attempt has been made to provide information that is both accurate and effective, the author does not assume any responsibility for the accuracy or use/misuse of this information.

Table of Contents

Chapter 1 – Introduction

If certain experts are to be believed, we are currently facing a crisis the likes of which we have never seen before; we are being faced with a global obesity epidemic.

Since 1980, the number of people suffering from obesity has literally more than doubled, with there being 1.4 billion overweight adults, and 500 million who can be considered as obese.

As far as children go, the numbers just keep on climbing, with certain countries seeing more than a quarter of their kids suffering from obesity. Long story short, if things keep on going the way they do, then in a few decades most of the world's population will be obese, if of course we even manage to survive that long. In order to fight this great plague it is important what it stems from... just like with any huge problem, there are numerous causes in play here.

For starters, we are leading increasingly sedentary lifestyles. Long gone are the days when we ploughed fields twelve hours a day or dug up coal in mines... long gone are the days when most people had to dedicate their working time to physical labor. These days, most people work sitting, or perhaps standing still, and needless to say, there isn't much effort involved in that, at least in a physical sense. The problem however is that even though we reduced our level of activity we kept on increasing how much we ate. As a result, our bodies simply aren't subjected to enough exercise to burn all the excess calories we gain, which leads to a noticeable weight gain. However, a lack of exercising coupled with overeating is not the only source of this problem.

Another cause for what we are observing today can be traced to economic fluctuations in regards to food prices. As it happens, in most cases, the cheaper a food is, the more filling and unhealthy it is. More specifically, the fast food industry is being referenced. Junk food restaurants have established themselves in countless poorer countries and economically-disadvantaged areas, providing people with cheap and fattening alternatives that allow them to save money. What's more, these alternatives are sometimes even tastier. In the end, the point is that the cost of healthy foods exceeds that of unhealthy ones.

Now with what we've just covered and as we begin this guide, it's important to realize that the world is in a bad state, health wise. But you don't have to accept what is happening in society. You are about to learn the 7 keys to transform your body and quite literally it will transform your life! So dive in, read, absorb and put into practise exactly what you learn here and see the change happen. You have the power in your hands to change your health and live the life you want to, rest assured that in the end, your body will thank you for it.

Key 1 - Must Eat Breakfast

When losing weight, most individuals would skip eating breakfast thinking that it is an effective method of eliminating weight. Now, what they do not realize is that this technique is not really effective and could even cause negative effects on their bodies. When dieting, one of the most important things to be aware of is the importance of eating breakfast.

Breakfast is referred to "breakfast" simply because it breaks the long fast. People are asleep during the night for many hours, so in the morning, it is necessary to eat something in order to feel better and have the energy to face the new day. More importantly, having breakfast is vital to a fat burning diet. If you want to lose weight fast, be mindful to eat breakfast every day.

Here are some of the reasons and importance of eating breakfast to the body when dieting:

• Breakfast will allow you to control your hunger and avoid eating snacks later on during the day. What would be the use of your diet when you would eventually eat more because you are hungry, since you skipped breakfast? If ever you skipped breakfast, just ensure to have a healthy snack so that you can still lose weight effectively.

• A healthy breakfast will aid in increasing your body's metabolism- Eating breakfast can actually boost one's metabolism. If you skip breakfast, you would tend to place your body into starvation mode and try to conserve energy that it can. Now, when you eat breakfast, you are also telling your body that you are awake and you are not fasting anymore. This means that your body is ready to burn fat and utilizes the energy during the day.

• A healthy breakfast would also help you consume enough calories- Having enough calories is essential because this is responsible in increasing your energy levels. When you regularly skip breakfast, you are also not consuming calories that would end up in dropping off of your energy levels. This would also slow down your metabolism. Losing weight would be that effective.

• Eating breakfast is essential in losing weight, as it helps the body attain its weight loss goal faster. According to research and studies, those individuals who miss breakfast are the ones who were 4 times more likely to be overweight. If you do not want to risk of gaining weight, ensure not to skip breakfast.

These are some of the importance of eating breakfast to the body when dieting. Breakfast is the most essential meal of the day; therefore, it is necessary not to skip it. Of course, when dieting, just make sure that you follow a healthy breakfast so that you can efficiently lose weight and achieve your weight loss goals.

Eating breakfast is good and healthy, so do not think that skipping breakfast would help you lose weight. This will just make you feel weak and unhealthy, and this will not do good with your goal of losing weight. Have a healthy breakfast every day and follow the right diet. In no time, you would be surprised to see the positive results with your health and body.

Drinking water plays a key role in dieting. If you ever find yourself stuck in a weight loss plateau despite following your diet program strictly, then it could be that you are not drinking enough water. Studies have shown that a lot people unsuspectingly suffer from severe or mild dehydration and you could be affected as well.

Your body requires water for various biochemical processes. The following are the benefits of drinking enough water to your body when dieting:

Water assists the body in the conversion of fat reserves into energy. When the body is dehydrated, the body's metabolism processes are slowed down and this impedes the breakdown of fats in the body, and in effect, your weight loss. If this happens, your weight loss curve hits a plateau.

Water holds naturally holds back your appetite. The hypothalamus region in your brain serves the role of controlling cravings and appetites, with the control centers for thirst and hunger situated next to one another. This means that drinking enough not only quenches your thirst, but it takes away the feelings of hunger as well. A study by Washington University found that drinking a glass of water before going to bed reduces mid-night cravings.

Water also helps in the prevention of sagging skin which is a common side effect of weight loss. It gives the skin a healthier and youthful look by helping in the reconstruction of destroyed skin cells.

Water assists in the elimination of waste products from the body. When dieting, the body loses weight and there are extra by products to be removed. This means that the body requires sufficient amounts of water into which the unwanted products will be dissolved and excreted from the body.

Water is effective in dealing with constipation. If the body does not get enough water, it is compelled to siphon it from its internal reserves, normally the colon, resulting into constipation. Normal bowel function will resume once the body receives adequate water.

In general, mild dehydration leads to a number of health complications. Mild dehydration is characterized by the following symptoms: fatigue, cravings, headaches and constipation. However, as soon as you get the water in balance, you achieve what diet experts refer to as a breakthrough point. At this point, as fluid retention in the body eases, the liver and endocrine systems start to operate more effectively, helping to reinstate your natural thirst, while reducing your cravings significantly. This eventually results into heightened metabolism rates which facilitate the breakdown and loss of fat in the body.

How Much Water Does the Body Need

In conclusion, the above benefits clearly show the importance of drinking water, particularly if you are on a diet. Nonetheless, everyone should make drinking water a habit. It should not only be done when you are thirsty as thirst, in itself, is an indication of the presence of dehydration. Hence, every adult ought to take at least eight glasses of water every day during cold weather. Since there is a lot of perspiration and loss of liquid during hot weather, additional glasses of water must be taken. Lastly, if exercises are part of your dieting plan, ensure that you drink 6-12 ounces of fluids after 15-20 intervals. This way, you will maintain the most favorable fluid balance during your exercises

KEY 3: PROPER SLEEP AND RECOVERY

To consider sleep as an activity is difficult. One assumes sleep to be a phase of inactivity or rest. But, the matter of fact is, that sleep is that active phase in our entire day's routine, when numerous bodily functions are expedited. The sales data of sleep inducing tranquilizers and sleeping pills prove the rising cases of sleep deficiency that owes a lot to the modern lifestyle. While profound research is available on the importance of exercise for the body, few embark on the desire to learn about rest and sleep...yet it is one of the most important factors in overall health and well-being.

What Is Sleep?

Firstly, it's important to understand that while the body rests , the mind and the brain go on a restorative hyper-drive. Bodily signals are sent to the various organs of to begin its build up for the next hour of optimum action. The more sleep deprived a person is, the more the chances of deficient physical and mental activity, as you've not allowed your body to recover from the previous bout or prepare for the next. Sleep is a period of nerve and muscle relaxation which begins a period of repair and rejuvenation of all the tissues and organs , much needed after a day of hectic often strenuous activity. Sleep is determined by a certain biological cycle called as the 'circadian clock'. It depends on the intervals of certain number of hours of being awake followed by sleep, and so on. Other elements affecting it could be- the amount of light, stress levels, metabolism levels and even the medication we may be taking.

The Power of Sleep

Sleep is a powerful energy booster owing to the fact that while we sleep the process called 'anabolism' gets underway; understood more simply as the recovery process for cells and tissues through the production of enzymes and proteins. It in fact counteracts the effect of 'catabolism' or the process that occurs as you exercise or work- out during the day which produces an action wherein energy is released from cells.This affects the molecular components of the body. If your catabolism exceeds anabolism ,little growth will happen . Thus those who strain themselves with a tougher workout or play an extra hour, must give their body the extra rest to sustain their growth of muscle mass, which is directly proportionate to fitness.
There is no contention to the fact that mental alertness,

concentration levels, communication, creativity, emotional balance and the productivity levels of an individual is also affected by the amount of sleep.

The Recovery Process

Prolonged sleep deprivation has been linked to anxiety and depression . Sleep induces the release of certain hormones that affect the central nervous system of the body thus affecting mood and emotional stability. Less sleep increases Cortisol which is a catabolic hormone and it decreases testosterone levels that are directly related to muscle mass gain. Less sleep also means a higher insulin level that increases your body's resistance to nutritional absorption.

While one can not contest the importance of fitness training including weight training one must understand the mechanics of what really happens to the body while this physical stress is being faced. While we exercise or lift weights, the muscle contracts or crunches thereby getting compressed or shortened.

This happens when the muscle microfibers compress. With every stimulus you give to your body, the muscle is strained to respond. What must however be realised is that between the phases of stimulus, the muscle needs to recover from it by building new bridges across the new muscle groups that are slowly forming. This growth is only possible when the body rests.

Another disturbing consequence that comes with compromising on the amount of sleep has is in the raised levels of cortisone which has been directly linked to more abdominal fats .While there has been encyclopedic quantum of research on the benefits of fitness programs, very little attention is paid to the importance of the body and its sleep requirement.

Balancing heavy workouts with its milder versions and adequate breaks from strenuous routines is not only the best antidote for perfect health, it's the best way to gain optimal benefits from your exercise routine

KEY 4 – HIGH INTENSITY CARDIO TO BURN FAT FASTER

Using high intensity cardio to burn fat faster is an approach that has been used by a number of people, it's benefits are huge and numerous, but it should always be done in a controlled environment and via a well set out plan. There is no doubt that this particular type of exercise does indeed burn fat a lot faster, but how does it actually work?

The reason why it works is because your body is being asked to produce a lot more energy than it has stored in order to deal with the intensity of the workout and it does this by burning off those fat reserves it has been keeping for a rainy day. Your body then has to keep producing energy even after you stop as it needs that in order to start repairing the muscles and settling your body after your strenuous workout.

It is also important to point out that this particular type of workout focuses on burning a different type of fat than what you would get doing a cardio workout that has a lower intensity such as a brisk walk. The problem with lower intensity cardio work is that it only gets your heart working to around 60% of the maximum heart rate, but this is not high enough for optimal fat burning in your body. Instead, you will only burn off the easy stuff, but the harder fat will still be there, so by increasing the intensity you burn off both types resulting in quicker weight loss.

There are other reasons why you should look at using this approach and one major reason is that you will then be able to deal with lactic acid a lot easier. It is this lactic acid build up that results in muscles becoming tired and burning with you then stopping, so by learning how to deal with this you can then workout for longer periods of time resulting in more calories and fat being burnt off and that weight disappearing.

This does take some time, but you at least know that whilst you are building up this resistance, your body is currently burning off fat as quickly as it needs to in order to give you energy to keep on working.

Finally, this approach results in improving the sensitivity of your body to insulin and the outcome of this is that the muscles are going to absorb the glucose, and use it to repair themselves and to get energy, rather than it being turned into fat stores. This does mean that when you burn off the fat, and then lose weight, it should stay that way rather than things fluctuating depending on how much exercise you have been doing during the week. Using high intensity cardio to burn fat faster does indeed work, but you must be prepared to put in a lot of work in order to achieve the best possible end result. By using this approach, your body will burn off fat as it needs that sudden surge of energy and you will also build lean muscle quicker so not only will you get fitter, but you will also notice a difference when you step on those scaled and this, after all, is the important part.

Key 5 – Learn How To Read Food Labels

In order for you to effectively experiment in your day to day eating and still choose nutritionally excellent foods, you must understand nutrition labels on packaging. Quite often the companies that manufacture different foods will claim on the packaging that they are low fat or healthy, but the truth of the matter is that there are hidden dangers in there for people that are on different diets. Being able to read the labels can, therefore, make a huge difference in the potential success of somebody that is trying to lose weight.

First, you must look at the serving size on the label because the nutritional information that is listed on there will tend to talk about a serving size that is smaller than the overall size of the item you are looking at. This is important because a number of companies will mention a portion of say 30g and list the nutritional information for that amount, but they know most people will take double so, in actual fact, it is then nowhere near as healthy as you think.

What you need to do is to look at the serving size and then, if you eat double, you must double those figures to see how healthy it actually is.

Another key area to look at is when they discuss the percentage of the daily recommended amount that a portion covers as this can tell you a lot about what is in the product and how it can affect your diet plan.

Yet again you need to look at the serving size along with this because if the serving size is 30g and it gives you 25% of your daily recommended allowance for salt and you take 60g, then you need to double this 25% in order to get a true reflection. Do also look to see if they mention how many calories per day this recommended amount is based on as the majority will be for 2000 calories, but you may be on less than that so you must calculate it accordingly.

Finally it is worth looking at how to read the individual ingredients as they will tend to use terms such as Sodium instead of salt or they will talk about carbohydrates instead of just listing how much sugar is in it. The thinking here is that by using more professional names, then it will sound healthier and it may be an idea to look at the names on labels you have near you now and make a note of the terms used so you know if unsaturated fats are good or bad, how much vitamin B12 is good for you and that you understand what type of sugar they have put into the food and what appears in it naturally due to the ingredients.

So that is how to read nutrition labels to help lose weight and there really is nothing complex about it as long as you just take your time to read things properly. By law they must have this information printed on there, so as long as you have an understanding of the amounts of different things you should eat for your diet plan, then you should find it that bit easier to go ahead and lose that weight.

KEY 6 – TONE YOUR BODY WITH RESISTANCE TRAINING

Excess weight is one of the most common problems that affect very many people from all across the globe. There is need to lose this unwanted weight so as to avoid health complications such as heart attack and other related diseases. In this chapter we will uncover resistance training exercises that can help you lose the excess fat. Examples of some of the common resistance training activities include weight lifting, sporting activities such as Basketball and Javelin, Isotonic resistance training which entails use of barbells and dumbbells. Below is a detailed guide of the importance of resistance training for losing weight.

Increase metabolic rate- The metabolic rate refers to the rate at which the body converts fats into energy for various purposes. Resistance training helps to increase the rate at which the fats are metabolized and this in turn helps to significantly reduce body fat.

Improves Body Posture- Since virtually all the physical activities in this category involves all the body muscles, they help to strengthen and increase muscles. This in turn helps one to improve body posture.

Increase Blood Circulation- For the body organs to operate optimally, they have to have sufficient and uninterrupted supply of blood rich in various nutrients such as proteins and carbohydrates. Resistance training helps to ensure that blood circulation in the body is optimal. This in turn helps to ensure that all vital body organs operate normally.

Decreases the Risk of Injuries- Losing weight involves a number of physical activities which may lead to injuries especially during the first stages. For example, new members might experience joint and muscles pains but this problem fades away as the body becomes acquainted to the activity. Resistance training will help decrease your susceptibility to injuries since the body parts will be able to withstand the pressure effectively.

Prevent cardiovascular diseases as well as Arthritis and diabetes- Excess weight has being closely linked to a number of health complications. Due to fact that these exercises will reduce and prevent accumulation of fats in the body, your chances of suffering from various cardiovascular diseases, diabetes and arthritis will be reduced significantly.

Boost Self Esteem- In most cases, persons suffering from excess weight problem are often stigmatized by the society. Fortunately, resistance training will help reduce this stigmatization and boost your self esteem.

Improves your Sleep Patterns- Excess weight can distort your sleeping pattern especially if the issue is stressing you too much. Through these physical activities, you will be able to solve this problem completely. This will in turn help you sleep much better at night as well as boost your productivity at home or at your work place.

Increase Bone Density and Strength- As the name suggest, this training will not only help you lose weight but also increase your bone density and strength. Increased bone strength will help reduce your susceptibility to injuries as well as enhance your performance of various physical tasks.

Be sure to consult a professional medical practitioner before enrolling in a particular program so as to avoid any health complications. Last but not least, ensure that your follow the instructions given by your trainer so as to achieve the full benefits from this training.

Common Misconceptions Of Resistance Training

1. Women who do strength training will become bulky and muscular

This myth has been around for so many years and unfortunately a lot of women believe it. Women do not have the ability to bulk up when they do resistance training exercises to increase their metabolism. Those who bulk up are the ones that take male hormones and inject anabolic steroids into their body. These kinds of women are mostly professional body builders. Therefore if you want to achieve that bulky look, it is very clear what you have to do. However, if you just want to achieve a lean toned body, resistance training exercises will give you just that; no bulky shoulders or arms.

2. Weights and expensive gym equipment are necessary for resistance training exercises

While free weights and other gym equipment are necessary to speed up your progress, they are not necessarily the only things that you can use to build muscles. There are a variety of ways that you can build muscle and some of them include: resistance bands, bar method, Pilate's, using your own body weight and isometric training. There are many programs for resistance training that do not use any equipment yet they help people to achieve excellent results.

3. When you grow old you cannot build muscle

This is not true because studies show that even people who are 70 years old can build muscle. In addition, people who are in their 50's or even 40's can be able to build adequate muscle mass with just a few training sessions per week.

4. Resistance training requires hours and hours of training per day

This takes the crown for being the biggest misconception about resistance training that can help boost your metabolism. Experts believe that as long as you eat a healthy well balanced diet and you do not have any diseases, you will only need about 20 minutes to half an hour sessions per week for you to realize results.

It is not the hours that you spend at the gym training but it is how often you do them and how hard you push your body. It has been established that when you add even a pound of muscle, your metabolism will increase and you can burn up to a maximum of 50 calories per day. Imagine how many calories you can burn when you add 10 pounds of muscle.

5. You will need to constantly lift heavy weights in order to maintain muscle mass

If you train every day you are likely to build more muscle and speed up your metabolism, right? Wrong! It has been proven that the people who achieve phenomenal results are the ones that take breaks in between their work out days. Muscles are built when our bodies are resting and not when they are active as most people would like to believe. The body also needs to recover after an intense work-out session.

KEY 7 – BODY TRANSFORMATION IS A LIFESTYLE

Whenever a special occasion or a holiday draws near, people often scramble for quick weight loss products or programs. While looking good in swimwear during summer is not a bad idea, looking for a short cut to weight loss can backfire. Truth is, weight loss is a lifestyle and not a fad. It is a result of a consistent effort that involves exercise, proper food intake, and the right amount of rest. This key will reveal how to achieve a healthy lifestyle that helps shed pounds permanently.

First, you have to change your perception about weight loss. It's not just a matter of watching your weight on the scale. Weight loss should be about changing your body composition by having less body fat and acquiring more muscles. For women, this means losing side handles and toning your thighs. For men, it mainly means decreasing your waist line. Lately, health experts are associating heart disease risks with a large waistline. Hence, having ripped abs is not just for aesthetic reasons but mainly for longevity. Weight loss is a goal to achieve good health; looking good should only be a consequence.

Second, you have to exercise on a daily basis if possible.

Start with brisk walking if you're overweight to prevent knee injuries. Perform this activity consistently by spending at least twenty minutes a day. Or, you can try a high intensity interval training (HIIT) to jumpstart your metabolism. Samples of which are burpees, bodysquats , push ups, and mountain climbers. This is way shorter to perform but requires cardiovascular health and lower body weight. It shocks the body to drastically increase metabolism that results to weight loss. However, this is not advisable for people who are just beginning to exercise.

Third, educate yourself on proper food intake. People who need to lose weight should consume less than their total energy expenditure. Plus, macronutrients like protein take centerstage along with complex carbohydrates. Reducing consumption of sugary food products does a lot of good to your body. Hyperlidimia, a condition where the body has high levels of cholesterol, is often triggered by obesity and diabetes.

Avoid eating fastfood. Prepare meals and bring them to work. Choose lean ground meat and season them with spices. Then, make sure you have a side dish of vegetables to add more fiber in your diet.

Lastly, minimize stress in your life by managing them. Again, you can resort to exercise to shake off stress from work. Listen to relaxing music. Enjoy time with your family or pursue a hobby you love. Stress produces hormones like cortisol that sabotage our attempts at weight loss. Also, get enough sleep so your mind and body can function optimally.

As you can see, weight loss is a lifestyle and not a fad. It means prioritizing exercise over a sedentary lifestyle. It means choosing the right food to fuel your body. Most of all, it means a healthy perspective of what life is all about - taking care of yourself for your loved ones

Conclusion: Tips To Begin The Transformation Today

As we close out this guide, we will cover a few extra tips and tricks that will help tremendously in transforming your body. Some tips might require you to adjust your lifestyle entirely. However, they are of great assistance in losing weight.

Exercise

It's the surest and most natural way to lose weight. Exercising can be done in so many ways to fit into your daily activities. For instance, you can decide to cycle to and from your work place or shopping center instead of taking a bus. On the other hand, you can opt to use the stairs instead of the elevator. Other activities like walking, jogging and running will also contribute to weight loss.

You can make exercising fun too, like playing basket ball with your peers or kids, going on long walks with your loved ones and many more fun activities that eventually will burn calories. On the other hand, you can structure an exercising routine every day that will involve at least 30 minutes of cardiovascular exercises.

Remember, exercises on top of burning up fat and calories also help in building a lean muscles mass which is essential for the body's metabolic rate.

Consume the right drinks

If it's not possible to quit alcohol entirely, limit yourself to a maximum of two on isolated cases when you have to take alcohol. Alcohol has no nutritional value to the body and the body usually uses it as its first energy source. Eventually, the food consumed ends up being stored as fat in the body. Alcohol also influences you to eat the wrong type of foods, preferably junk foods that are high in calories. It's, therefore, essential to avoid alcohol consumption, or to limit its consumption, as much as possible.

Similarly, avoid fruit drinks and soda. Instead opt for diet drinks and plenty of water. Water suppresses the regular urges to eat and consequently help you lose some weight. It also keeps the body hydrated, which is ideal for nutrients' release to the body.

Green tea is also favorite beverage for people on a weight loss program. Studies have demonstrated that consuming green tea leads to more calories being burnt faster than those who do not consume it.

Consume the right foods

Eat the right foods that will not contribute to weight gain but rather to weight loss. Grape fruit has been found effective in helping people lose weight. Consuming half a grape fruit three times a day burns more calories by boosting the body's metabolism. On the other hand, avoid or minimize on the consumption of fats, especially animal fats as they are high in cholesterol. Opt for skim milk and low fat cheese. Similarly, consume lean meat, preferably white meat. In addition, opt for unprocessed foods as their calories and fat content is lower. On the other hand, if you have to consume processed food, like bread, opt for the whole grain bread as its high in dietary fiber content. Fiber assists in burning calories.

Also things to avoid are, refined sugar containing products and junk food. Look for sugar substitutes to use in the place of sugar. Junk food is low in nutritional value and high in calories content. Avoid it as well. However, ensure you consume plenty of fruits and vegetables and minimize on starch products for an almost ideal body weight.

9 781973 914358